The Road through Recovery

A fight Against brain cancer and tumour

Finley Peyton

Copyright

No part of this book should be copied, reproduced without the author's permission @2024

Contents

Copyright 3
Introduction 6
Chapter one 11
What is Brain Cancer? 11
Chapter 3 15
What is Brain Tumor? 15
Chapter 4 42
Types of Brain Cancer 42
Chapter 5 62
Causes of Brain Cancer 62
Chapter 6 79
Brain Cancer in Kids 79
Chapter 7 88
Brain Cancer in Adults 88
Chapter 8 96
Ways To Prevent Brain Cancer 96
Chapter 9 101
Living With People With Brain Cancer 101
Chapter 10 107
Treatment 108
Chapter 11 115
Remedy 115
Herbal Remedy 120

Introduction

Brain cancer refers to the presence of malignant tumors in the brain or central spinal cord. These tumors can arise from the brain tissue itself (primary brain tumors) or spread to the brain from other parts of the body (metastatic brain tumors). The complexity of the brain's structure and function makes brain cancer particularly challenging to diagnose and treat.

Types of Brain Cancer

Brain tumors are classified into two main categories:

Primary Brain Tumors: These originate in the brain. They can be further classified based on the type of cells involved:

Gliomas: Tumors that arise from glial cells, which support and protect neurons. This category includes astrocytomas, oligodendrogliomas, and glioblastomas, the latter being one of the most aggressive forms.

Meningiomas: Tumors that develop from the meninges, the protective membranes surrounding the brain and spinal cord. They are usually benign but can cause significant pressure on brain structures.

Acoustic Neuromas: Benign tumors that develop on the vestibular nerve, which connects the inner ear to the brain, often leading to hearing loss and balance issues. 2.

Metastatic Brain Tumors: These tumors originate from cancer cells that have spread to the brain from other parts of the body, such as the lungs, breasts, or skin. Metastatic brain tumors are more common than primary brain tumors in adults.

Symptoms

The symptoms of brain cancer can vary widely based on the tumor's size, location, and growth rate. Common symptoms include: -
Headaches that may worsen over time
Seizures
Nausea and vomiting
Changes in vision, hearing, or speech
Cognitive and personality changes
Weakness or numbness in limbs
Balance and coordination issues

Diagnosis

Diagnosing brain cancer typically involves several steps:
Medical History and Symptoms Review: A thorough assessment of the individual's medical history and presenting symptoms.

Neurological Examination: A series of tests to evaluate brain function, including reflexes, coordination, and cognitive abilities.

Imaging Studies: Techniques such as magnetic resonance imaging (MRI) or computed tomography (CT) scans are essential for visualizing tumors and determining their location and size.

Biopsy: A definitive diagnosis often requires a biopsy, where a tissue sample is taken from the tumor for pathological examination.

Treatment

Treatment for brain cancer is highly individualized and may include a combination of:
Surgery: To remove the tumor or obtain a biopsy.
Radiation Therapy: To target and kill cancer cells, especially after surgery to eliminate residual cells.

Chemotherapy: Systemic treatment using drugs to kill cancer cells or inhibit their growth.

Targeted Therapy and Immunotherapy: Emerging treatments that focus on specific characteristics of cancer cells or enhance the immune response against tumors.

Prognosis

The prognosis for brain cancer varies significantly based on several factors, including the tumor type, location, grade, and the patient's overall health. Some brain tumors are more responsive to treatment than others, and early diagnosis can significantly improve outcomes.

Brain cancer is a complex and challenging condition that requires a multidisciplinary approach for effective management. Advances in research continue to improve understanding, diagnosis, and treatment options, offering hope for better outcomes for individuals diagnosed with this serious illness. Ongoing support and comprehensive care are essential for patients and their families throughout the cancer journey.

Chapter one

What is Brain Cancer?

Brain cancer refers to the presence of malignant tumors in the brain, which can arise from the brain tissue itself or from other parts of the body through metastasis. Tumors in the brain can be categorized as primary or secondary.

Primary brain tumors originate in the brain, while secondary brain tumors, also known as metastatic tumors, occur when cancer cells spread from other parts of the body to the brain. There are various types of primary brain tumors, which are classified based on the type of cells involved. Some common types include:

1. Gliomas: These tumors develop from glial cells, which support and protect neurons. Gliomas include astrocytomas, oligodendrogliomas, and glioblastomas, the latter being the most aggressive form.

2. Meningiomas: These tumors arise from the meninges, the protective membranes surrounding the brain and spinal cord. Meningiomas are often benign but can cause problems due to their location.

3. Pituitary Tumors: These tumors occur in the pituitary gland at the base of the brain and can affect hormonal balance in the body.

4. Medulloblastomas: These are common in children and develop in the cerebellum, affecting balance and coordination.

5. Ependymomas: These tumors arise from ependymal cells lining the ventricles of the brain and can block the flow of cerebrospinal fluid.

Symptoms of brain cancer can vary widely depending on the tumor's location and size. Common symptoms include headaches, seizures, changes in vision or hearing, difficulty with balance or coordination, and cognitive changes such as memory loss or confusion. Diagnosis typically involves a combination of neurological examinations, imaging studies like MRI or CT scans, and sometimes a biopsy to confirm the presence of cancer cells. Treatment options often include surgery, radiation therapy, and chemotherapy, and the choice of treatment depends on the type and stage of the tumor, as well as the patient's overall health. Research into brain cancer is ongoing, focusing on understanding the genetic and molecular basis of tumors, developing targeted therapies, and improving treatment outcomes for patients

Chapter 3

What is Brain Tumor?

A brain tumor is an abnormal growth of cells within the brain or central spinal canal. These tumors can be classified as either primary, originating in the brain, or secondary (metastatic), which are cancers that have spread to the brain from other parts of the body. The nature of brain tumors can vary widely in terms of their type, growth rate, and treatment options.

Types of Brain Tumors

Primary Brain Tumors:

-Gliomas: This category includes astrocytomas, oligodendrogliomas, and glioblastomas. Glioblastoma multiforme (GBM) is the most aggressive form and is known for rapid growth and poor prognosis.

-Meningiomas: Typically benign, these tumors arise from the meninges, the protective membranes surrounding the brain and spinal cord. They often grow slowly and may not cause symptoms initially.

-Pituitary Tumors: These tumors occur in the pituitary gland and can affect hormone levels, leading to various systemic effects.

-Neurocytomas: These are rare tumors that can affect the ventricular system of the brain.

Secondary Brain Tumors: - These tumors are a result of cancer spreading to the brain from other areas, such as the lungs, breast, skin, or colon. The treatment and prognosis depend on the primary cancer type and its stage.

Symptoms

The symptoms of brain tumors can vary significantly depending on the size, type, and location of the tumor. Common symptoms include:
Headaches that may worsen over time
Seizures
Nausea and vomiting
Changes in vision, hearing, or speech
Weakness or numbness in limbs
Cognitive changes, including memory problems or personality shifts
Difficulty with balance or coordination

Diagnosis

Diagnosing a brain tumor typically involves several steps:
Neurological Exam:

A neurological exam is a crucial part of the diagnostic process for brain cancer. This examination helps assess the function of the brain and nervous system, allowing healthcare providers to identify any abnormalities that may indicate the presence of a brain tumor or other neurological conditions. The exam typically involves several components, each aimed at evaluating different aspects of neurological function.

Components of a Neurological Exam
Patient History: - The clinician begins by gathering a detailed medical history, including the patient's symptoms, duration of symptoms, any previous neurological issues, family history of cancer, and other relevant medical conditions.
2. Mental Status Examination: - This part assesses cognitive function, including attention, memory, language, and reasoning abilities. The healthcare provider may ask the patient to: -

Repeat a series of words or numbers. - Solve simple math problems. - Describe their understanding of concepts or follow multi-step commands.

3. Cranial Nerve Examination: - The cranial nerves are tested to evaluate sensory and motor functions related to the head and neck. This includes: -
Vision: Checking visual acuity, peripheral vision, and response to light. –

Pupillary Response: Assessing the size and reaction of pupils to light. –

Eye Movement: Evaluating the ability to track moving objects and check for any nystagmus (involuntary eye movements). –

Facial Sensation: Testing sensation in different areas of the face and checking for facial symmetry.

Hearing: Assessing auditory function and balance.

4. Motor Function: - The strength and coordination of limbs are evaluated. The clinician may ask the patient to: -

Squeeze their hands. - Raise their arms and legs against resistance. - Perform coordinated movements like touching their fingers to their nose or heel-to-shin testing.

5. Sensory Examination: - This assesses the patient's ability to feel sensations such as light touch, pain, temperature, and vibration. The clinician may use a pinprick, cotton swab, or tuning fork to test different sensory modalities.

6. Reflex Testing: - Deep tendon reflexes (e.g., knee and ankle jerks) are evaluated to assess the integrity of the spinal cord and peripheral nerves. Abnormal reflexes may indicate neurological dysfunction.

7. Gait and Balance Assessment: - The patient's ability to walk and maintain balance is observed. The clinician may ask the patient to walk in a straight line, perform heel-to-toe walking, or stand on one foot to evaluate balance and coordination.

8. Postural Stability: - The clinician may assess the patient's ability to maintain stability while standing still or during movement.

Interpretation of Findings

The results of the neurological exam can provide valuable information about the location and extent of a potential brain tumor. Abnormal findings may suggest specific areas of the brain that are affected by a tumor, including: -
Cognitive Impairments: Difficulty with memory, attention, or language may indicate tumors in areas responsible for cognitive processing. –
Motor Weakness: Weakness or coordination problems could suggest lesions in the motor cortex or pathways. –
Sensory Changes: Alterations in sensation may indicate involvement of the sensory cortex or peripheral nerves. –

Visual Disturbances: Changes in vision can be linked to tumors affecting the optic pathways or occipital lobe.

A thorough neurological exam is essential for evaluating patients suspected of having brain cancer. It provides critical insights into neurological function and helps guide further diagnostic imaging and treatment decisions. If abnormalities are found during the exam, additional tests such as MRI or CT scans may be ordered to confirm the presence of a brain tumor and determine its characteristics

Imaging Studies: Imaging studies play a vital role in the diagnosis, evaluation, and management of brain tumors. These non-invasive techniques allow healthcare providers to visualize the brain's structure, identify abnormalities, and assess the tumor's characteristics. The most commonly used imaging modalities for brain tumors include:

-Magnetic Resonance Imaging (MRI) MRI is the gold standard for brain tumor imaging due to its high resolution and ability to provide detailed images of brain anatomy. –

-Technique: MRI uses powerful magnets and radio waves to produce detailed images of the brain. Different sequences (e.g., T1, T2, FLAIR) can highlight various tissue characteristics. –

Advantages: -

-Excellent soft tissue contrast, making it highly effective for differentiating between normal brain tissue and tumors. –

-Ability to visualize edema (swelling), which is often associated with tumors. –

-Functional MRI (fMRI) can assess brain activity and map critical areas of function, helping guide surgical planning. –

-Use in Diagnosis: MRI can confirm the presence of a tumor, determine its size and location, and evaluate its relationship to surrounding structures. It is also useful for monitoring treatment response and detecting recurrence.

-Computed Tomography (CT) Scan CT scans are often used as a preliminary imaging tool, especially in emergency settings. –

-Technique: CT uses X-ray technology to create cross-sectional images of the brain. Contrast agents may be administered intravenously to enhance visualization.

Advantages:

-Rapid acquisition of images, making it useful in acute situations. –

Effective for identifying bleeding, calcifications, and bone abnormalities.

-Use in Diagnosis: CT scans can help detect the presence of a tumor, especially in patients with acute neurological symptoms. However, they provide less detail than MRI for soft tissue differentiation.

1) Positron Emission Tomography (PET) Scan PET scans can provide functional information about brain tumors by

highlighting areas of increased metabolic activity. –

2)Technique: PET scans involve injecting a radioactive tracer, often fluorodeoxyglucose (FDG), which is taken up by metabolically active cells, including tumor cells. –

Advantages:

Helps differentiate between tumor recurrence and radiation necrosis by assessing metabolic activity.

Can provide information about tumor grading and aggressiveness based on metabolic activity.

Use in Diagnosis: PET scans are typically used in conjunction with MRI or CT to provide additional information about a brain tumor's metabolic characteristics and to evaluate treatment response.

Magnetic Resonance Spectroscopy (MRS) MRS is an advanced MRI technique that provides biochemical information about brain tissue. –

Technique: MRS detects the concentrations of specific metabolites in the brain, allowing for analysis of the chemical composition of tumors.

Advantages:

Can help differentiate between tumor types and assess tumor grade based on metabolic profiles.

Useful for monitoring treatment response by evaluating changes in metabolite levels.

Use in Diagnosis: MRS is often used to complement conventional MRI findings, providing additional insights into tumor biology.

Diffusion Tensor Imaging (DTI) DTI is a specialized MRI technique that maps the white matter tracts in the brain. –

Technique: DTI assesses the diffusion of water molecules in brain tissue, providing visualizations of white matter integrity and connectivity. –

Advantages:

Helps identify pathways that may be affected by tumors, aiding in surgical planning and preserving critical brain functions. –

Use in Diagnosis: DTI can be particularly useful for assessing brain tumors located near vital white matter tracts, guiding neurosurgeons during resection.

Imaging studies are essential tools in the diagnosis and management of brain tumors. MRI is the most widely used imaging modality due to its superior soft tissue contrast and ability to provide detailed anatomical information. CT scans, PET scans, MRS, and DTI also play important roles in evaluating tumors, guiding treatment decisions, and monitoring responses to therapy. Together, these imaging techniques contribute to a comprehensive understanding of brain tumors, facilitating accurate diagnosis and effective management.

Biopsy: A biopsy of a brain tumor is a crucial diagnostic procedure that involves the extraction of a tissue sample from the tumor for histopathological examination. This process helps determine the tumor's type, grade, and molecular characteristics, which are essential for guiding treatment decisions and predicting prognosis.

Types of Brain Tumor Biopsies

There are several methods for obtaining a biopsy from a brain tumor, each suited to different clinical situations:

Stereotactic Biopsy: -

Technique: This minimally invasive procedure uses advanced imaging techniques (such as CT or MRI) to precisely locate the tumor. A hollow needle is then inserted through a small incision in the scalp to obtain a tissue sample. –

Advantages:

Stereotactic biopsy is less invasive than open surgery, has a lower risk of complications, and can be performed on tumors that are difficult to access. It allows for targeted sampling of the tumor while minimizing damage to surrounding brain tissue.

Use: This method is often employed for deep-seated tumors or when the tumor is located near critical brain structures, making surgical resection more challenging.

Open Biopsy: -

Technique: An open biopsy involves surgical removal of a portion of the tumor or the entire tumor through a larger incision in the skull (craniotomy). This procedure may be performed if the tumor is accessible and if resection is anticipated.

Advantages:

Provides a larger tissue sample, which can be beneficial for more accurate diagnosis and comprehensive analysis. In some cases, the entire tumor may be removed during the procedure, leading to therapeutic benefits.

Use: Typically indicated when the tumor is located in an area that is amenable to surgical access and when a more extensive evaluation is nenecessary

Endoscopic Biopsy: -

Technique: This technique utilizes an endoscope, a thin tube with a camera and instruments, to access and biopsy the tumor through natural openings or small incisions. It is often used for tumors located in the ventricular system or near the base of the skull. –

Advantages:

Minimally invasive, with reduced recovery time and lower risk of complications. –

Use: Suitable for certain types of tumors that can be accessed through the endoscopic approach.

Procedure Overview

Regardless of the biopsy method employed, the general process typically includes:

Preoperative Assessment: - Patients undergo imaging studies (CT or MRI) to determine the tumor's location and plan the biopsy approach. A thorough medical history and physical examination are also conducted.

Anesthesia: - Biopsies are usually performed under general anesthesia to ensure patient comfort and immobility during the procedure.

Tissue Sample Collection: - The chosen method (stereotactic, open, or endoscopic) is performed to obtain the tissue sample, with care taken to minimize damage to surrounding brain tissue.

Post-Procedure Care: - After the biopsy, patients are monitored for any complications, such as bleeding or infection. Recovery protocols vary based on the biopsy type and extent of the procedure.

Histopathological Evaluation

Once the tissue sample is obtained, it is sent to a pathology laboratory for detailed examination. The analysis typically includes: -

Microscopic Examination: Pathologists assess the tissue for cellular characteristics, patterns of growth, and signs of malignancy. –

Tumor Grading: Tumors are graded based on their aggressiveness, with higher grades indicating more aggressive behavior. –

Molecular Testing: Additional tests may be performed to identify specific genetic mutations or markers that can guide targeted therapies.

Conclusion

A biopsy is a critical step in the diagnosis and management of brain tumors. It provides essential information about the tumor's type, grade, and potential behavior, which is vital for developing an effective treatment plan. The choice of biopsy method depends on various factors, including the tumor's location, size, and the patient's overall health. By obtaining a definitive diagnosis, biopsies facilitate personalized treatment approaches and improve patient outcomes.

Treatment Options

Treatment for brain tumors depends on several factors, including the tumor type, location, size, and the patient's overall health. Common treatment modalities include:

Surgery: The primary goal is to remove as much of the tumor as possible. In some cases, complete resection may not be feasible due to the tumor's location or involvement with critical brain structures.

Radiation Therapy: This is often used post-surgery to target any remaining tumor cells or as a primary treatment for inoperable tumors. Stereotactic radiosurgery (SRS) uses focused radiation beams to treat small tumors.

Chemotherapy: Systemic treatments may be used to target tumor cells, particularly in aggressive tumors like glioblastomas. Newer targeted therapies and immunotherapies are also being explored.

Palliative Care: For patients with advanced disease or poor prognosis, palliative care focuses on improving quality of life and managing symptoms.

Prognosis

The prognosis for brain tumor patients varies widely based on tumor type, grade, location, and the patient's overall health. While some benign tumors can be effectively treated with surgery alone, aggressive tumors like glioblastomas often have a more challenging prognosis. Ongoing research is essential for improving treatment outcomes and understanding the biological mechanisms underlying brain tumors.

Research and Future Directions

Research into brain tumors is continually evolving, with a focus on: -

Genetic and Molecular Profiling: Understanding the genetic mutations and molecular characteristics of tumors can lead to personalized treatment approaches. - Novel Therapeutics: Investigating new drugs, including targeted therapies and immunotherapies, holds promise for improving outcomes. -Clinical Trials: Participation in clinical trials offers patients access to cutting-edge treatments and contributes to the advancement of knowledge in brain tumor management. In summary, brain tumors are complex disorders that require a multidisciplinary approach for diagnosis and treatment. Ongoing research and advancements in medical science continue to enhance understanding and improve patient outcomes.

Brain tumors encompass a diverse and intricate group of conditions that can significantly impact individuals' health and quality of life. Understanding the various aspects of brain tumors involves exploring their biology, clinical manifestations, treatment strategies, and ongoing research initiatives.

Biology of Brain Tumors

Brain tumors arise from the uncontrolled growth of cells in the brain or surrounding tissues. The biological characteristics of these tumors are crucial in determining their behavior, treatment response, and prognosis.

Cell Types: Brain tumors can originate from different types of cells, including: -
Neurons: Nerve cells that can give rise to neuroblastomas or other neuronal tumors. –
Glial Cells: These are supportive cells in the brain, and tumors arising from them are called gliomas. Types include: -
Astrocytomas: Derived from astrocytes, they vary from low-grade to aggressive forms such as glioblastomas. –
Oligodendrogliomas: These tumors originate from oligodendrocytes and

often have a better prognosis than astrocytomas. –

Ependymal Cells: Tumors from these cells are called ependymomas and can occur in the ventricles of the brain.

Tumor Grading: Brain tumors are graded based on their histological characteristics, which indicate how aggressive they are: -

Low-Grade Tumors: Typically slow-growing and less aggressive (e.g., grade I and II). They may be more amenable to surgical resection. –

High-Grade Tumors: More aggressive and fast-growing (e.g., grade III and IV). Glioblastomas are grade IV tumors known for rapid progression. Symptoms and Diagnosis The symptoms of brain tumors vary widely and can be influenced by the tumor's size, location, and growth rate. Common symptoms include: -

Focal Neurological Deficits: Weakness, numbness, or coordination problems depending on the tumor's location. –

Cognitive Changes: Memory loss, confusion, or personality changes. - Seizures: New-onset seizures can often be the first sign of a brain tumor. – Increased Intracranial Pressure: Symptoms such as headaches, nausea, and vomiting can occur due to swelling or blockage of cerebrospinal fluid (CSF) flow.

Diagnostic Techniques

Diagnosing brain tumors typically involves a combination of clinical evaluation and imaging studies:

Imaging Studies: -

Magnetic Resonance Imaging (MRI): This is the gold standard for visualizing brain tumors, providing detailed images of the brain's anatomy and the tumor's characteristics. –

Computed Tomography (CT) Scans: Useful in emergency settings to quickly assess for bleeding or major structural changes.

Biopsy: - A definitive diagnosis often requires obtaining a tissue sample through a biopsy, which can be performed during surgery or using minimally invasive techniques. The histopathological examination of the tumor helps determine its type and grade. Treatment Strategies The treatment of brain tumors is multifaceted and tailored to the individual patient based on tumor type, location, and overall health.

Common treatment modalities include:

Surgery: - Surgical resection is often the first-line treatment for accessible tumors. The goal is to remove as much of the tumor as possible while preserving surrounding healthy tissue. In some cases, complete removal may not be feasible, especially for tumors located near critical brain structures.

Radiation Therapy: - Radiation can be used as an adjuvant therapy following surgery to target residual tumor cells.

Chemotherapy: - Chemotherapeutic agents may be used, particularly for aggressive tumors like glioblastomas. Temozolomide is a commonly used oral chemotherapy drug that has shown efficacy in treating certain brain tumors.

Targeted Therapy and Immunotherapy: - Emerging treatments focus on targeting specific molecular pathways or utilizing the immune system to attack tumor cells. Research in this area is rapidly evolving, with numerous clinical trials underway.

Palliative Care: - For patients with advanced disease or poor prognosis, palliative care plays a crucial role in managing symptoms and improving quality of life.

Research and Future Directions

The field of brain tumor research is dynamic, with ongoing efforts aimed at improving understanding and treatment:

Genetic Research: - Understanding the genetic mutations associated with different brain tumors is critical for developing targeted therapies. Biomarkers are being identified to predict treatment response and prognosis.

nnovative Therapies: - New therapeutic approaches, including CAR T-cell therapy and oncolytic virus therapy, are being explored in clinical trials. These innovative treatments aim to harness the body's immune response against tumors.

Patient-Centered Research: - Increasing emphasis is being placed on quality of life and survivorship in research, recognizing the importance of psychosocial support and rehabilitation for patients and families.

Brain tumors represent a complex group of conditions that require a comprehensive understanding of their biology, clinical presentation, and treatment options. Advances in research and technology continue to improve diagnosis and therapeutic strategies, offering hope for better outcomes and quality of life for patients. Continued advocacy for awareness and funding is essential to further enhance the understanding and treatment of brain tumors.

Chapter 4

Types of Brain Cancer

Brain cancer encompasses a variety of tumor types that can arise from different cells within the brain or surrounding structures. The classification of brain tumors can be complex, but they are generally categorized into primary and secondary (metastatic) tumors. Here are the main types of brain cancer:

Primary Brain Tumors

Gliomas: Gliomas are a type of brain tumor that arises from glial cells, which are the supportive cells of the central nervous system. They account for a significant proportion of primary brain tumors and can vary widely in terms of their characteristics, behavior, and response to treatment. Gliomas are classified based on the type of glial cell from which they originate, as well as their grade, which indicates how aggressive the tumor is.

Types of Gliomas
Astrocytomas: -
Origin: Derived from astrocytes, star-shaped glial cells that support and protect neurons. –
Grades: -
Grade I: Pilocytic astrocytoma, typically benign and slow-growing, often found in children. –

Grade II: Low-grade astrocytoma, can be more aggressive over time. –

Grade III: Anaplastic astrocytoma, a malignant and aggressive form. –

Grade IV: Glioblastoma multiforme (GBM), the most aggressive form of astrocytoma with a poor prognosis.

Oligodendrogliomas: -

Origin: Arise from oligodendrocytes, which produce the myelin sheath that insulates nerve fibers. –

Grades: -

Grade II: Low-grade oligodendroglioma, typically slow-growing. –

Grade III: Anaplastic oligodendroglioma, more aggressive and malignant. –

Genetic Features: Often associated with specific genetic mutations, including 1p/19q co-deletion, which can influence treatment response and prognosis.

Ependymomas: -

Origin: Ependymal cells that line the ventricles of the brain and the central canal of the spinal cord. –

Grades: -

Grade II: Ependymoma, with potential for recurrence. –

Grade III: Anaplastic ependymoma, a more aggressive form. –

Location: Commonly found in children and can occur in various locations, including the spinal cord.

Mixed Gliomas: - These tumors contain a combination of glial cell types, such as both astrocytic and oligodendrocytic components. An example is anaplastic oligoastrocytoma, which can have varying degrees of aggressiveness.

Symptoms

The symptoms of gliomas depend on their size, location, and growth rate. Common symptoms may include: -

Headaches: Often persistent and may worsen over time. –

Seizures: New-onset seizures are common in glioma patients. –

Cognitive Changes: Memory problems, confusion, or personality changes may occur. –

Motor or Sensory Deficits: Weakness, numbness, or coordination issues can arise depending on the tumor's location.
—

Increased Intracranial Pressure: Symptoms such as nausea, vomiting, and vision changes may result from swelling or blockage of cerebrospinal fluid (CSF) flow.

Diagnosis

Diagnosing gliomas typically involves:

1. Neurological Examination: Assessing neurological function and symptoms.
2. Imaging Studies: MRI is the primary imaging modality used to visualize the tumor, its size, and its location.
3. Biopsy: A tissue sample is often obtained to confirm the diagnosis and determine the tumor type and grade through histopathological examination.

Treatment

The treatment approach for gliomas varies based on the tumor's type, grade, and location, as well as the patient's overall health. Common treatment modalities include:

1. Surgery: The primary treatment for gliomas is surgical resection, aiming to remove as much of the tumor as possible while preserving surrounding brain tissue. Complete resection is more feasible for low-grade tumors.

2. Radiation Therapy: Often used as an adjuvant treatment following surgery to target residual tumor cells. Stereotactic radiation therapy may be employed for precision targeting.

3. Chemotherapy: Systemic treatments, such as temozolomide, are commonly used, especially for high-grade gliomas like glioblastomas. Chemotherapy is often combined with radiation therapy.

4. Targeted Therapy and Immunotherapy: Emerging therapies focus on specific genetic mutations or immune responses to treat gliomas. Research is ongoing to identify effective targeted treatments.

Prognosis

The prognosis for glioma patients varies widely depending on the tumor type, grade, location, and the patient's age and overall health. Low-grade gliomas generally have a better prognosis than high-grade gliomas, such as glioblastomas, which are associated with a poorer outcome. Advances in treatment and ongoing research continue to improve understanding and management strategies for gliomas, offering hope for better outcomes for affected individuals.
Ependymomas: These arise from ependymal cells lining the ventricles of the brain or spinal cord. They can occur in both children and adults and may be benign or malignant.

Meningiomas: Meningiomas are a type of brain tumor that arises from the meninges, the protective membranes covering the brain and spinal cord. These tumors are typically considered extra-axial, meaning they originate outside the brain tissue itself. Meningiomas are among the most common types of primary brain tumors in adults and can vary significantly in terms of their behavior, symptoms, and treatment options.

Characteristics of Meningiomas
Types: - Meningiomas can be classified into several types based on their histological features: -
Benign (Grade I): The majority of meningiomas are benign and grow slowly. They often have well-defined borders and may not invade surrounding tissues. –
Atypical (Grade II): These tumors show some features of malignancy and have a higher risk of recurrence after treatment. –
Anaplastic (Grade III): These are malignant meningiomas that grow more rapidly and have a higher potential for invasion and metastasis.

Location: - Meningiomas can occur in various locations within the central nervous system, including:

Convexity Meningiomas: Located on the outer surface of the brain. –

Sphenoid Wing Meningiomas: Found near the base of the skull. –

Falx Cerebri Meningiomas: Situated along the midline between the two hemispheres of the brain. –

Intradural Meningiomas: These can extend into the spinal canal and affect the spinal cord.

Symptoms

The symptoms of meningiomas depend on their size and location, as well as the extent to which they affect surrounding brain structures. Common symptoms may include: -

Headaches: Often persistent and may worsen over time. –

Seizures: New-onset seizures can occur, especially if the tumor irritates the brain. –

Neurological Deficits: Depending on the tumor's location, symptoms may include weakness, sensory changes, or coordination problems. –

Vision Changes: Tumors near the optic nerve can cause visual disturbances or loss of vision. –

Cognitive Changes: Memory problems, confusion, or personality changes may arise, particularly with larger tumors.

Diagnosis

The diagnosis of meningiomas typically involves:

1. Neurological Examination: A thorough assessment of neurological function and symptoms is conducted.

2. Imaging Studies: MRI is the preferred imaging modality for visualizing meningiomas. CT scans may also be used, especially in emergency settings.

3. Biopsy: In some cases, a biopsy may be performed to confirm the diagnosis and determine the tumor's grade.

Treatment

The treatment approach for meningiomas depends on various factors, including the tumor's size, location, symptoms, and whether it is benign or malignant. Common treatment options include:

1. Observation: Small, asymptomatic meningiomas may be monitored with regular imaging, especially if they are not causing significant symptoms or neurological deficits.

2. Surgery: Surgical resection is often the primary treatment for symptomatic meningiomas. The goal is to remove as much of the tumor as possible while preserving surrounding brain tissue. Complete resection is associated with a better prognosis.

3. Radiation Therapy: This may be used as an adjunct to surgery, particularly for tumors that cannot be fully removed or for atypical and anaplastic meningiomas. Techniques such as

stereotactic radiosurgery can target the tumor precisely.

4. Chemotherapy: While not commonly used for meningiomas, it may be considered in cases of aggressive or recurrent tumors, especially those that are anaplastic.

Prognosis

The prognosis for individuals with meningiomas varies based on factors such as tumor grade, location, and completeness of surgical resection. Benign meningiomas generally have a favorable prognosis, with low rates of recurrence after complete removal. Atypical and anaplastic meningiomas, on the other hand, have a higher risk of recurrence and may require more aggressive treatment approaches. In summary, meningiomas are common brain tumors that arise from the meninges. They can range from benign to malignant and present with various symptoms depending on their size and location. Diagnosis typically involves imaging studies and, in some cases, biopsy. Treatment options include observation, surgical resection, and radiation therapy, with the prognosis generally being favorable for benign tumors. Ongoing research continues to enhance understanding and treatment strategies for meningiomas.

Acoustic Neuromas (Vestibular Schwannomas): Acoustic neuromas, also known as vestibular schwannomas, are benign tumors that develop on the vestibulocochlear nerve, which is the eighth cranial nerve responsible for hearing and balance. These tumors arise from Schwann cells, which provide insulation and support for nerve fibers. Although classified as benign, acoustic neuromas can cause significant symptoms due to their location and pressure on adjacent structures.

Characteristics of Acoustic Neuromas

Incidence: - Acoustic neuromas are relatively rare, with an estimated incidence of about 1 in 100,000 people per year. They are most commonly diagnosed in adults, typically between the ages of 30 and 60.

Growth Patterns: - These tumors grow slowly, often over several years, and may remain small without causing symptoms. However, as they grow, they can exert pressure on surrounding nerves and brain structures.

Location: - Acoustic neuromas typically occur at the cerebellopontine angle, where the cerebellum meets the brainstem. This location is crucial as it affects both auditory and balance functions.

Symptoms

Symptoms of acoustic neuromas usually develop gradually and may vary depending on the size of the tumor and its impact on nearby structures. Common symptoms include: -

Hearing Loss: Often the first symptom, typically unilateral (affecting one ear). The hearing loss may be gradual and can range from mild to profound. —
Tinnitus: Ringing or buzzing in the affected ear is a common complaint. —
Balance Issues: Patients may experience dizziness or a sensation of unsteadiness due to the tumor's effect on the vestibular portion of the nerve. —
Facial Weakness or Numbness: As the tumor grows, it may compress the facial nerve (cranial nerve VII), leading to facial weakness or altered sensation. —
Headaches: While less common, headaches may occur due to increased intracranial pressure if the tumor grows large enough.

Diagnosis

The diagnosis of acoustic neuromas typically involves several steps:
Neurological Examination: A thorough assessment of hearing, balance, and facial function is conducted.

Imaging Studies: MRI is the preferred imaging modality for detecting acoustic neuromas. It provides detailed images of the brain and can reveal the presence, size, and extent of the tumor. In some cases, a CT scan may be used, particularly if MRI is contraindicated.

Audiometric Testing: Hearing tests are performed to evaluate the extent of hearing loss and to assess the function of the auditory nerve.

Treatment

The treatment approach for acoustic neuromas depends on several factors, including the tumor's size, growth rate, the patient's age, overall health, and the presence of symptoms. Common treatment options include:

Observation: For small, asymptomatic tumors, a "watch and wait" approach may be adopted. Regular MRI scans are conducted to monitor the tumor for any changes in size or symptoms.

Surgery: Surgical removal of the tumor is often recommended for larger tumors or those causing significant symptoms. The goal is to remove as much of the tumor as possible while preserving hearing and facial nerve function. The two main surgical approaches are:

Translabyrinthine Approach: This approach is often used for larger tumors and involves removing the inner ear structures to access the tumor. –

Retrosigmoid Approach: This method allows for preservation of hearing in some cases and involves accessing the tumor through the back of the skull.

Radiation Therapy: Stereotactic radiosurgery (such as Gamma Knife or CyberKnife) is a non-invasive treatment option used to target the tumor with highly focused radiation beams. This approach is often considered for tumors that are not amenable to surgery or for patients who prefer to avoid surgical intervention.

Prognosis

The prognosis for individuals with acoustic neuromas is generally favorable, particularly for benign tumors. Many patients experience significant improvement in symptoms after treatment, especially if the tumor is removed successfully. Hearing preservation is possible in some cases, particularly with the retrosigmoid surgical approach or when using radiation therapy. However, some patients may still experience residual symptoms, such as tinnitus or balance issues, even after treatment. In conclusion, acoustic neuromas are benign tumors arising from the vestibulocochlear nerve, leading to symptoms primarily related to hearing and balance. Diagnosis typically involves imaging studies and audiometric testing, while treatment options vary based on tumor size and symptoms. With appropriate management, patients can achieve good outcomes and maintain a reasonable quality of life. Ongoing research continues to enhance understanding and treatment strategies for acoustic neuromas.

4. Pituitary Tumors: These tumors arise from the pituitary gland and can be either benign (adenomas) or malignant. They can affect hormone levels, leading to various endocrine disorders.

5. Medulloblastomas: Primarily seen in children, these malignant tumors usually arise in the cerebellum. They are known for their aggressive behavior and potential to spread within the central nervous system.

6. Choroid Plexus Tumors: These tumors originate from the choroid plexus, which produces cerebrospinal fluid. They can be benign or malignant and are more common in children.

7. Primary CNS Lymphoma: A type of non-Hodgkin lymphoma that occurs in the brain and central nervous system. It is more common in individuals with weakened immune systems.

Secondary Brain Tumors (Metastatic Brain Tumors)

Secondary brain tumors are not originally from the brain but have spread to it from other parts of the body. Common sources of metastatic brain tumors include:

Lung Cancer: The most common source of metastatic brain tumors.

Breast Cancer: Frequently spreads to the brain.

Melanoma: Known for being aggressive and often metastasizing to the brain.

Kidney Cancer: Can also spread to the brain.

Colorectal Cancer: Less common but can result in metastatic brain tumors.

Understanding the types of brain cancer is crucial for diagnosis and treatment planning. Each tumor type has distinct characteristics, including growth patterns, treatment responses, and prognoses. Ongoing research continues to improve knowledge of these tumors, leading to better treatment options and outcomes for patients diagnosed with brain cancer.

Chapter 5

Causes of Brain Cancer

The exact causes of brain cancer are not fully understood, but several risk factors and potential causes have been identified through research. These factors may contribute to the development of brain tumors, although having one or more of these factors does not guarantee that a person will develop brain cancer. The following are some of the known and suspected causes and risk factors:

Genetic Factors: Certain inherited genetic syndromes increase the risk of brain tumors. Conditions such as neurofibromatosis type 1 and type 2, Li-Fraumeni syndrome, and tuberous sclerosis are linked to a higher incidence of brain cancer.

Brain cancer can arise from a combination of genetic and environmental factors. Some of the key genetic factors that have been identified as contributing to the development of brain tumors include:

Inherited Genetic Syndromes: Certain hereditary conditions increase the risk of brain cancer. For example, individuals with Neurofibromatosis type 1 (NF1) and type 2 (NF2), Li-Fraumeni syndrome, and Turcot syndrome have a higher predisposition to developing gliomas and other types of brain tumors.

Oncogenes: Mutations in specific genes that promote cell growth can lead to tumor formation. For instance, mutations in the EGFR (epidermal growth factor receptor) gene are common in glioblastoma, a highly aggressive form of brain cancer. Similarly, alterations in the PDGFRA (platelet-derived growth factor receptor alpha) gene can also contribute to tumor growth.

Tumor Suppressor Genes: Genes that normally help prevent uncontrolled cell growth can also play a role when mutated. The TP53 gene, which encodes the p53 protein involved in cell cycle regulation and apoptosis, is frequently mutated in various brain tumors, including gliomas. Another important tumor suppressor is the PTEN gene, whose loss is associated with increased risk of glioblastoma.

Chromosomal Abnormalities: Brain tumors often exhibit specific chromosomal alterations. For example, the 1p/19q co-deletion is a common finding in oligodendrogliomas and is associated with a better prognosis.

Epigenetic Changes: Beyond DNA mutations, changes in gene expression regulation without altering the DNA sequence can also contribute to brain cancer. Methylation patterns that silence tumor suppressor genes can promote tumorigenesis.

Family History: A family history of brain tumors may suggest a genetic predisposition, although most brain tumors occur sporadically without a clear hereditary link. Understanding these genetic factors is essential for developing targeted therapies and improving treatment outcomes for patients with brain cancer.

The relationship between genetic factors and brain cancer is complex and multifaceted, involving a range of genetic mutations, chromosomal abnormalities, and inherited syndromes.

Here are some of the key aspects that further elaborate on this connection:

Genetic Mutations and Pathways Brain tumors often result from mutations in genes that are critical in regulating cell growth, division, and survival. Some notable pathways involved include:

PI3K/AKT/mTOR Pathway: This signaling pathway is often altered in brain tumors, particularly in glioblastomas. Mutations in the PTEN gene, which negatively regulates this pathway, can lead to uncontrolled cell proliferation.

Ras Pathway: The RAS family of oncogenes (such as KRAS and NRAS) can become mutated, leading to increased cell growth and division. This pathway is often implicated in various cancers, including brain tumors.

Cell Cycle Regulation: Genes that control the cell cycle, such as CDKN2A and RB1, when mutated, can lead to loss of cell cycle control, allowing for the development and progression of tumors.

Specific Tumor Types and Their Genetic Profiles Different types of brain tumors exhibit distinct genetic alterations:

Glioblastoma: This aggressive tumor is characterized by mutations in the EGFR gene, loss of PTEN, and alterations in the TP53 gene. The presence of the IDH1 mutation is also significant in lower-grade gliomas and secondary glioblastomas.

Oligodendroglioma: These tumors often show 1p/19q co-deletion, which is a hallmark of this tumor type and is associated with better responses to chemotherapy and radiation.

Medulloblastoma: This pediatric brain tumor has several subtypes, each with different genetic alterations. For example, the WNT subtype often has mutations in the CTNNB1 gene, while the SHH subtype may involve mutations in the PTCH1 or SUFU genes.

Environmental Factors and Genetic Interactions While genetic predisposition plays a critical role, environmental factors can also influence the risk of developing brain cancer. These factors might interact with genetic susceptibility, such as: -

Ionizing Radiation: Exposure to high doses of radiation, such as from previous cancer treatments, is a well-established risk factor for brain tumors.

Chemical Exposures: Certain chemicals, like those used in the production of rubber and pesticides, have been investigated for potential links to brain cancer, although findings are often inconclusive.

Research and Future Directions
Ongoing research aims to better understand the genetic landscape of brain tumors. Techniques such as whole-genome sequencing and targeted gene panels are being used to identify novel mutations and pathways involved in tumorigenesis. This knowledge is crucial for developing personalized medicine approaches, where treatments are tailored based on the specific

genetic alterations present in a patient's tumor.

Genetic Counseling and Testing For individuals with a family history of brain tumors or related genetic syndromes, genetic counseling and testing can be beneficial. Identifying mutations can provide valuable information about the risk of developing brain cancer and help in surveillance and management strategies. In conclusion, the genetic factors associated with brain cancer involve a complex interplay of mutations, inherited syndromes, and environmental influences. As our understanding of these factors grows, it holds promise for improving prevention, diagnosis, and treatment strategies for brain tumors.

Environmental Exposures: Exposure to ionizing radiation, particularly during medical treatments for other conditions, is a well-established risk factor for developing brain cancer. Occupations that involve exposure to certain chemicals or pesticides may also contribute to risk, although the evidence is not as strong.

Environmental factors can significantly influence the risk of developing brain cancer, although the exact mechanisms are often complex and not fully understood. Here are some of the main environmental factors that have been associated with an increased risk of brain tumors:

Ionizing Radiation Exposure to ionizing radiation is one of the most well-established environmental risk factors for brain cancer. This includes:

Medical Treatments: Patients who receive radiation therapy for other cancers, particularly in the head and neck region, have an increased risk of developing secondary brain tumors later in life.

Nuclear Accidents: Incidents like the Chernobyl disaster have been linked to an increased incidence of brain tumors in populations exposed to radioactive fallout.

Chemical Exposure Certain chemicals have been investigated for their potential links to brain cancer, although findings are often mixed. Some notable exposures include:

Pesticides: Some studies suggest that exposure to specific pesticides may be associated with an increased risk of brain tumors. For example, agricultural workers exposed to organophosphate pesticides may have a higher risk.

Industrial Chemicals: Chemicals such as formaldehyde, vinyl chloride, and some solvents used in industrial settings have been studied for potential associations with brain cancer.

Occupational Exposures Certain professions may carry an increased risk of brain cancer due to exposure to harmful substances or environments. Occupations that have been studied include:

Agriculture: Farmers and agricultural workers may be at higher risk due to pesticide exposure and other chemical agents.

Manufacturing and Construction: Workers in these fields may be exposed to various chemicals, solvents, and heavy metals that could potentially increase cancer risk.

Electromagnetic Fields (EMF) The potential link between exposure to electromagnetic fields, particularly from mobile phones and power lines, has been a topic of research. While some studies suggest a possible association with brain tumors, particularly gliomas and acoustic neuromas, the evidence remains inconclusive and debated within the scientific community.

Infections Certain viral infections have been linked to an increased risk of brain tumors:

Epstein-Barr Virus (EBV): There is evidence suggesting a potential association between EBV and certain types of brain tumors, particularly in immunocompromised individuals.

Human Immunodeficiency Virus (HIV): Individuals with HIV/AIDS are at a higher risk for primary central nervous system lymphoma, a type of brain cancer.

Lifestyle Factors While lifestyle factors are primarily associated with other types of cancer, there may be indirect links to brain cancer risk:

Diet and Nutrition: Some studies suggest that diets low in fruits and vegetables may contribute to cancer risk, although specific links to brain cancer are less clear.

Obesity: Obesity has been associated with various cancers, and while the direct link to brain cancer is less well established, it may contribute to overall cancer risk.

Age and Gender Although not strictly environmental factors, age and gender can influence cancer risk. Brain tumors are more common in children and older adults, and some types are more prevalent in males than females. In summary, while genetics play a crucial role in brain cancer development, environmental factors also contribute significantly to the risk. Ongoing research aims to clarify these relationships and better understand how environmental exposures might interact with genetic predispositions to influence brain tumor development.

3. Age: Brain cancer can occur at any age, but certain types of tumors are more common in specific age groups. For instance, medulloblastomas are more prevalent in children, while glioblastomas are more frequently diagnosed in adults.

4. Gender: Some studies suggest that males may be at a slightly higher risk of developing brain tumors compared to females, although this varies by tumor type.

5. Family History: A family history of brain tumors may increase an individual's risk, indicating that genetic predisposition may play a role. However, most brain cancer cases occur in individuals without a family history of the disease.

6. Immune System Disorders: Individuals with weakened immune systems, such as those with HIV/AIDS or those who have undergone organ transplants, may have a higher risk of developing brain tumors.

7. Previous Cancer: Survivors of certain types of cancer, particularly childhood cancers, may have an increased risk of developing brain tumors later in life, often as a result of prior treatments like radiation.

While these factors are associated with an increased risk of brain cancer, it is important to note that ongoing research continues to explore other potential causes, including viral infections and lifestyle factors. However, as of now, no definitive lifestyle-related causes have been established. Understanding the causes of brain cancer remains a crucial area of research, as it may lead to better prevention strategies and treatments.

Symptoms of Brain Cancer

The symptoms of brain cancer can vary widely depending on the tumor's location, size, and the rate at which it grows. They may develop gradually or appear suddenly. Some common symptoms include:

1. Headaches: Persistent or worsening headaches that may be different from typical headaches are often one of the first signs. These headaches may be

more severe in the morning or may wake a person from sleep.

2. Seizures: New-onset seizures can occur in individuals who have not previously had them. The type and frequency of seizures can vary based on the tumor's location.

3. Cognitive Changes: Patients may experience memory problems, difficulty concentrating, confusion, or changes in personality. These cognitive changes can be subtle at first but may become more pronounced over time.

4. Vision and Hearing Problems: Tumors located near the optic nerves or auditory pathways can lead to blurred vision, double vision, or hearing loss. Some individuals may also experience visual field deficits.

5. Balance and Coordination Issues: Tumors affecting the cerebellum or

brainstem can result in difficulty with balance, coordination, and fine motor skills. Individuals may experience dizziness or a sensation of being unsteady.

6. Weakness or Numbness: Depending on the location of the tumor, individuals may experience weakness or numbness in specific areas of the body. This may manifest as difficulty using an arm or leg.

7. Nausea and Vomiting: Increased intracranial pressure caused by a tumor can lead to nausea and vomiting, particularly in the morning.

8. Fatigue: Unexplained or excessive fatigue is a common symptom that may accompany other neurological issues.

9. Changes in Sensation: Patients may experience altered sensations, such as

tingling or a loss of feeling in certain parts of the body.

10. Hormonal Changes: Tumors affecting the pituitary gland can lead to hormonal imbalances, resulting in various symptoms, such as changes in menstrual cycles or unusual growth patterns. These symptoms can be caused by various medical conditions, not just brain cancer. Therefore, it is essential for individuals experiencing any of these symptoms, especially if they are persistent or worsening, to seek medical evaluation. Early diagnosis and treatment can significantly impact outcomes for individuals with brain tumors.

Chapter 6

Brain Cancer in Kids

Brain cancer in children is a serious and complex condition that differs significantly from brain cancer in adults, both in terms of types of tumors and treatment responses. Pediatric brain tumors are the most common solid tumors in children and the second most common type of childhood cancer overall, following leukemia. Here's an overview of brain cancer in children, including its types, symptoms, diagnosis, treatment, and prognosis.

Types of Brain Cancer in Children

Pediatric brain tumors can be classified into various types, with some of the most common including:

Medulloblastomas: These are the most common type of malignant brain tumor in children, typically arising in the cerebellum. They often spread to other parts of the central nervous system but are treatable with a combination of surgery, radiation, and chemotherapy.

Gliomas: This group includes various types of tumors originating from glial cells. In children, common types include:

Pilocytic Astrocytoma: Usually benign and slow-growing, often found in the cerebellum or optic nerve.
Diffuse Intrinsic Pontine Glioma (DIPG): A highly aggressive tumor located in the brainstem, known for its poor prognosis.

Ependymomas: Tumors that arise from ependymal cells lining the ventricles of the brain or spinal cord. They can occur in various locations and may be challenging to treat.

Craniopharyngiomas: Typically benign tumors located near the pituitary gland, they can affect hormone levels and cause various symptoms due to their location.

Choroid Plexus Tumors: These tumors form in the choroid plexus, a structure that produces cerebrospinal fluid. They can be either benign or malignant.

Symptoms

The symptoms of brain cancer in children can vary based on the tumor's location and size. Common symptoms may include:
Persistent headaches, often worse in the morning or accompanied by vomiting

Nausea and vomiting
Changes in vision or double vision
Seizures
Difficulty with balance or coordination
Cognitive or behavioral changes, such as personality shifts or decreased academic performance
Weakness or numbness in limbs

Diagnosis

Diagnosing brain cancer in children typically involves several steps:

Medical History and Physical Examination: Initial assessments include a review of symptoms and a neurological examination.

Imaging Studies: Magnetic resonance imaging (MRI) is the primary imaging technique used to identify and locate tumors in the brain.

Biopsy: A biopsy may be performed to obtain tissue samples for pathological examination, confirming the tumor type and grade.

Treatment

The treatment for pediatric brain cancer is highly individualized and may include:

Surgery: Often the first line of treatment, surgery aims to remove as much of the tumor as possible while preserving surrounding brain tissue.

Radiation Therapy: Used post-surgery or when surgery isn't feasible, radiation can target remaining cancer cells and reduce tumor size.

Chemotherapy: This may be used in conjunction with surgery and radiation, particularly for certain types of tumors like medulloblastomas.

Targeted Therapy and Clinical Trials: Ongoing research into new treatments may provide additional options for children with brain tumors, particularly those that are difficult to treat with conventional methods.

Prognosis

The prognosis for children with brain cancer varies widely based on several factors, including:
The type, location, and grade of the tumor.
The child's age and overall health.
How well the tumor responds to treatment.
Some pediatric brain tumors have favorable outcomes, especially when diagnosed and treated early, while others, like DIPG, carry a more challenging prognosis.

Support and Care

Caring for a child with brain cancer involves not only medical treatment but also emotional and psychological support for both the child and their family. This includes:

Psychosocial Support: Access to counseling and support groups can help families navigate the emotional challenges of a cancer diagnosis.

Rehabilitation Services: Physical, occupational, and speech therapy may be necessary to aid recovery and improve the child's quality of life post-treatment.

Educational Support: Schools can provide accommodations to support the child's learning needs during and after treatment.

Brain cancer in children presents unique challenges and complexities that require a comprehensive, multidisciplinary approach to treatment and care. Advances in research and treatment options continue to improve outcomes for pediatric patients, offering hope for better management and survival rates. Ongoing support from healthcare providers, family, and community resources is essential in helping children and their families cope with the journey of cancer care.

Chapter 7

Brain Cancer in Adults

Brain cancer in adults encompasses a range of malignant tumors that originate in the brain or central nervous system. These tumors can be classified as primary, arising from brain tissue, or secondary, where cancer spreads to the brain from other parts of the body. Understanding brain cancer in adults involves examining its types, symptoms, diagnostic methods, treatment options, and prognosis.

Types of Brain Cancer in Adults

Gliomas: These tumors arise from glial cells and are the most common type of primary brain tumor in adults. They include:

Astrocytomas: Ranging from low-grade (slow-growing) to high-grade (aggressive), glioblastoma multiforme (GBM) is the most aggressive form of astrocytoma.

Oligodendrogliomas: Typically slower-growing tumors that can also be aggressive, often arising in the cerebral hemispheres.

Ependymomas: Tumors that develop from ependymal cells lining the ventricles of the brain and spinal cord.

2. Meningiomas: These are usually benign tumors that arise from the meninges, the protective membranes surrounding the brain and spinal cord. While often slow-growing, they can still cause significant pressure on brain structures.

3. Acoustic Neuromas (Vestibular Schwannomas): Benign tumors that develop on the vestibular nerve, affecting balance and hearing. They can lead to hearing loss, tinnitus, and balance issues.

4. Pituitary Tumors: These can be benign (adenomas) or malignant and affect hormone levels, potentially leading to various endocrine disorders.

Metastatic Brain Tumors: These tumors originate from cancer that has spread to the brain from other parts of the body, such as the lungs, breast, or skin. Metastatic brain tumors are more common than primary brain tumors in adults.

Symptoms

Symptoms of brain cancer in adults can vary widely depending on the tumor's location, size, and growth rate. Common symptoms include:

Persistent headaches, often worsening over time or occurring in specific patterns

Seizures, which may be the first sign of a brain tumor

Nausea and vomiting

Cognitive changes, including memory problems, difficulty concentrating, or personality changes

Vision or hearing changes, such as blurriness or hearing loss

Weakness or numbness in limbs

Coordination and balance issues

Diagnosis

Diagnosing brain cancer typically involves several steps:

Medical History and Physical Examination: A thorough assessment of symptoms and neurological function.

Imaging Studies: Magnetic resonance imaging (MRI) is the most common imaging technique used to identify and locate tumors. Computed tomography (CT) scans may also be used.

Biopsy: Obtaining a tissue sample from the tumor to determine the type and grade of cancer is often essential for a definitive diagnosis.

Treatment

Treatment for brain cancer in adults is highly individualized and may involve a combination of approaches:

Surgery: The primary goal is to remove as much of the tumor as possible while preserving normal brain function. In some cases, complete removal is not feasible due to the tumor's location.

Radiation Therapy: This is often used post-surgery to eliminate remaining cancer cells or as a primary treatment for inoperable tumors. Techniques such as stereotactic radiosurgery may be employed for precision targeting.

Chemotherapy: Systemic treatment using drugs to kill cancer cells or inhibit their growth. Chemotherapy may be used alone or in conjunction with surgery and radiation.

Targeted Therapy and Immunotherapy: Emerging treatments that focus on specific genetic mutations or enhance the immune response against cancer cells are being explored in clinical trials.

Prognosis

The prognosis for brain cancer in adults varies widely based on several factors, including:
The type and grade of the tumor
The location of the tumor in the brain
The age and overall health of the patient
The response to treatment

Some brain tumors, such as low-grade gliomas, may have better outcomes compared to aggressive tumors like glioblastomas, which have a poorer prognosis despite treatment.

Support and Care
Caring for adults with brain cancer involves not only medical treatment but also support for emotional and psychological well-being. Important aspects include:
Psychosocial Support: Access to counseling services and support groups can help patients and their families cope with the emotional impact of a brain cancer diagnosis.

Rehabilitation Services: Physical, occupational, and speech therapy may be necessary to assist with recovery and improve quality of life after treatment.

Palliative Care: This approach focuses on relieving symptoms and improving the quality of life for patients with advanced disease.

Brain cancer in adults is a complex condition that requires a multidisciplinary approach for effective management. Advances in research continue to improve understanding, diagnosis, and treatment options, providing hope for better outcomes. Ongoing support for patients and their families is essential throughout the cancer journey, addressing both the physical and emotional challenges presented by the disease.

Chapter 8

Ways To Prevent Brain Cancer

While there is no guaranteed way to prevent brain cancer, certain lifestyle choices and risk management strategies may help reduce the risk of developing the disease. Here are several approaches that can contribute to overall brain health and potentially lower the risk of brain cancer:

1. Avoiding Ionizing Radiation: Limiting exposure to ionizing radiation, particularly from medical imaging, is crucial. If possible, discuss with healthcare providers the necessity of scans that involve radiation, such as CT

scans, and consider alternatives when appropriate.

2. Healthy Diet: A well-balanced diet rich in fruits, vegetables, whole grains, and lean proteins can support overall health. Some studies suggest that diets high in antioxidants and anti-inflammatory foods may help protect against various cancers.

3. Regular Exercise: Engaging in regular physical activity can help maintain a healthy weight and improve overall health. Exercise has been associated with a reduced risk of several types of cancer.

4. Avoiding Tobacco and Limiting Alcohol: Smoking is a known risk factor for many cancers, including some brain tumors. Avoiding tobacco and limiting alcohol consumption can contribute to overall cancer prevention.

5. Protecting Against Environmental Toxins: Reducing exposure to potential carcinogens in the environment, such as certain chemicals and pesticides, may lower risk. This can include proper ventilation when using chemicals and following safety guidelines in occupational settings.

6. Managing Hormonal Factors: For women, hormonal changes and treatments may influence cancer risk. Discussing hormone replacement therapy with a healthcare provider can help assess risks and benefits.

7. Regular Health Check-ups: Routine medical check-ups can help identify health issues early. Discuss any neurological symptoms with a healthcare provider promptly, as early detection of potential issues can lead to better outcomes.

8. Genetic Counseling: For individuals with a family history of brain tumors or genetic syndromes associated with increased cancer risk, genetic counseling may provide valuable information and help in making informed decisions regarding monitoring and preventive strategies.

9. Maintaining Mental Health: Stress management and mental wellness are important for overall health. Practices such as mindfulness, meditation, and engaging in social activities can support mental well-being.

10. Staying Informed: Keeping up-to-date with the latest research on brain cancer and understanding personal risk factors can empower individuals to make informed health choices. While these strategies cannot guarantee prevention, they can contribute to a healthier lifestyle and may reduce the risk of brain cancer and other diseases.

It's important for individuals to consult with healthcare professionals regarding their specific health needs and risk factors.

Chapter 9

Living With People With Brain Cancer

Caring for someone with brain cancer requires a compassionate and supportive approach, as individuals may experience a range of physical, emotional, and cognitive challenges throughout their journey. Here are several ways to provide effective care and support:

1. Understand Their Condition -
Educate Yourself: Learn about brain cancer, its symptoms, treatment options, and potential side effects. Understanding the condition can help

you empathize with the patient's experiences and anticipate their needs.

Offer Emotional Support –
Be Present: Sometimes, just being there for the individual can provide immense comfort. Listen actively, allowing them to express their feelings, fears, and concerns without judgment.

Encourage Open Communication: Create a safe space for them to talk about their emotions and experiences. Validate their feelings and encourage them to share their thoughts.

Assist with Daily Activities-
Help with Routine Tasks: Depending on their condition, they may need assistance with daily activities such as cooking, cleaning, and personal hygiene. Offer to help with these tasks, but also encourage independence when possible.

Transportation: Offer to drive them to medical appointments, therapy sessions, or support groups, as they may experience fatigue or cognitive challenges that make driving difficult.

Manage Symptoms and Side Effects-

Monitor Symptoms: Keep track of any changes in their condition, including physical symptoms like headaches, nausea, or mood changes. Report these to their healthcare team.

Support Treatment Side Effects: Help manage side effects of treatments such as fatigue, nausea, or pain. This may include preparing nutritious meals, suggesting relaxation techniques, or helping them follow medical advice.

Encourage Healthy Habits –

Nutrition: Provide healthy meals that are easy to prepare and eat. Focus on nutrient-dense foods that can support their immune system and overall health.

Hydration: Encourage them to stay hydrated, as this is important for overall health and can help manage side effects.

Promote Physical Activity –

Gentle Exercise: If they are able, encourage light physical activity, such as walking or stretching. Gentle exercise can help improve mood, increase energy, and enhance overall well-being.

Create a Comfortable Environment –

Modify Living Space: Ensure their home environment is safe and comfortable. This may involve removing trip hazards, providing comfortable seating, and creating a quiet, peaceful atmosphere.

Foster a Routine: Establishing a daily routine can provide stability and predictability, which can be comforting for someone facing uncertainty.

Provide Social Interaction –

Encourage Socialization: Help them stay connected with family and friends. Arrange visits, phone calls, or virtual meetings to combat feelings of isolation.

Engage in Activities: Participate in activities they enjoy, whether it's watching movies, reading, or engaging in hobbies that can be done together.

Seek Professional Help –

Palliative Care: Consider involving a palliative care team, which specializes in providing relief from symptoms and improving quality of life for individuals with serious illnesses.

Counseling Services: Encourage them to seek professional counseling or support groups to help navigate the emotional challenges of their diagnosis.

Take Care of Yourself –

Self-Care: Caring for someone with brain cancer can be emotionally and physically demanding. Make sure to take time for yourself, engage in activities you enjoy, and seek support when needed.

Set Boundaries: It's important to establish boundaries to prevent caregiver burnout. Recognize your limits and seek help from others when necessary.

Caring for someone with brain cancer involves a blend of emotional support, practical assistance, and promoting overall well-being. By fostering a compassionate and understanding environment, you can significantly enhance the quality of life for the individual while also taking care of your own needs as a caregiver. Open communication and collaboration with healthcare professionals are essential components of effective caregiving.

Chapter 10

Treatment

The treatment for brain cancer varies based on several factors, including the type and grade of the tumor, its location, the patient's overall health, and personal preferences. Treatment options often involve a combination of therapies to achieve the best outcomes. Here are the primary treatment modalities for brain cancer:

1. Surgery-
Surgery is often the first line of treatment for many types of brain tumors, especially when the tumor is accessible and can be safely removed. The goals of surgery include:

Tumor Removal: The primary objective is to excise as much of the tumor as possible without damaging surrounding healthy brain tissue. Complete removal can lead to better outcomes.

Biopsy: If the tumor cannot be fully removed, a biopsy may be performed to obtain a tissue sample for diagnosis.

Decompression: In cases where the tumor is causing increased intracranial pressure, surgery may relieve pressure on the brain.

2.Radiation Therapy-

Radiation therapy uses high-energy rays to target and kill cancer cells. It can be employed in various scenarios:

Post-Surgery Treatment: Following surgery, radiation is often used to eliminate any remaining tumor cells, particularly for high-grade tumors.

Primary Treatment: For inoperable tumors or when surgery is not feasible, radiation may serve as the primary treatment.

Stereotactic Radiosurgery: This highly focused form of radiation allows for the delivery of a precise dose of radiation to the tumor while minimizing exposure to surrounding healthy tissue.

Chemotherapy-
Chemotherapy involves the use of drugs to kill cancer cells or inhibit their growth. It is often used in specific situations:
Adjunct Therapy: Chemotherapy may be used alongside surgery and radiation to enhance treatment efficacy, particularly for aggressive tumors like glioblastomas.

Oral or Intravenous Administration: Depending on the specific drugs used, chemotherapy can be administered orally or via intravenous infusion.

Targeted Chemotherapy: Certain drugs target specific genetic mutations within tumor cells, providing a more tailored approach to treatment.

Targeted Therapy-
Targeted therapy involves drugs that specifically target molecular changes in cancer cells. These treatments aim to interfere with cancer cell growth and survival by focusing on specific pathways. Examples include:
Bevacizumab (Avastin): This drug inhibits angiogenesis, the formation of new blood vessels that tumors need to grow. It is used in certain types of brain tumors, particularly glioblastomas.

Molecularly Targeted Agents: Research is ongoing into various agents that target specific genetic mutations, such as EGFR mutations.

Immunotherapy-

Immunotherapy aims to harness the body's immune system to fight cancer. This approach is still being studied in brain cancer but shows promise:

Checkpoint Inhibitors: These drugs help the immune system recognize and attack cancer cells.

Vaccines: Experimental vaccines are being developed to stimulate an immune response against specific tumor antigens.

Clinical Trials-

Participation in clinical trials may offer access to new and experimental treatments that are not yet widely available. Clinical trials can provide opportunities to receive cutting-edge therapies and contribute to research that may benefit future patients.

Supportive Care-

In addition to these primary treatments, supportive care plays a vital role in managing symptoms and improving quality of life. This can include:

Symptom Management: Addressing pain, nausea, seizures, and other neurological symptoms through medications and therapies.

Rehabilitation: Physical, occupational, and speech therapy may be necessary to help patients regain function and adapt to changes resulting from the tumor or treatment.

The treatment of brain cancer is highly individualized, and a multidisciplinary approach is often employed, involving neurosurgeons, oncologists, radiation therapists, and supportive care teams. Early diagnosis and timely intervention are crucial for improving outcomes. If diagnosed with brain cancer, it is essential for patients to discuss treatment options, potential side effects, and prognosis with their healthcare providers to make informed decisions tailored to their specific circumstances.

Chapter 11

Remedy

While there are no known "remedies" for brain cancer in the sense of a guaranteed cure outside of established medical treatments, various complementary and supportive approaches can play a role in managing symptoms, improving quality of life, and supporting overall well-being during conventional treatment. It is important to note that these approaches should not replace standard medical therapies, but they may be used alongside them as part of a comprehensive care plan. Here are some supportive strategies that individuals may consider:

1. Nutritional Support-

A well-balanced diet can help support overall health and may enhance the effectiveness of conventional treatments. Some dietary considerations include:

Antioxidant-Rich Foods: Incorporating fruits and vegetables high in antioxidants may help combat oxidative stress. Foods such as berries, leafy greens, and nuts are beneficial.

Omega-3 Fatty Acids: Found in fish, flaxseeds, and walnuts, omega-3s may have anti-inflammatory properties.

Hydration: Staying well-hydrated is essential for overall health and can help manage side effects of treatment.

2. Complementary Therapies-

Various complementary therapies may help alleviate symptoms and improve quality of life:

Acupuncture: Some patients find relief from pain, nausea, and anxiety through acupuncture, which involves the insertion of thin needles at specific points on the body.

Massage Therapy: Therapeutic massage can help reduce tension, alleviate pain, and promote relaxation.

Yoga and Meditation: Both practices can improve mental well-being, reduce stress, and enhance quality of life. Mindfulness techniques may also help manage anxiety and depression.

3. Psychological Support-
Mental health support is vital for individuals facing a brain cancer diagnosis. Considerations include:
Counseling or Therapy: Professional counseling can provide emotional support and coping strategies.

Support Groups: Connecting with others who have experienced similar challenges can offer comfort and understanding.

Mind-Body Techniques-

Mind-body approaches can promote relaxation and improve emotional well-being:

Mindfulness and Meditation: These practices focus on present-moment awareness and can help reduce stress and anxiety.

Breathing Exercises: Simple breathing techniques can promote relaxation and help manage stress.

Herbal and Natural Supplements-

Some individuals explore herbal supplements or natural products to support health. However, it is crucial to consult with a healthcare provider before starting any supplements, as they can interact with conventional treatments or have side effects. Popular options include:

Turmeric (Curcumin): Known for its anti-inflammatory properties, curcumin is being studied for its potential effects on cancer.

Green Tea: Contains antioxidants and polyphenols that may have protective effects.

Palliative Care-

Palliative care focuses on providing relief from the symptoms and stress of serious illness. It aims to improve quality of life for both the patient and their family. This approach can be integrated at any stage of treatment and can include:

Pain Management: Effective strategies to manage pain and discomfort.

Symptom Control: Addressing side effects from treatments, such as nausea or fatigue.

While there is no known alternative remedy for brain cancer, supportive and complementary approaches can play a significant role in enhancing quality of life and managing symptoms. It is essential for individuals with brain cancer to work closely with their healthcare team to create a holistic treatment plan that incorporates both conventional and supportive therapies. Always discuss any new treatments, supplements, or therapies with a healthcare professional to ensure safety and appropriateness.

Herbal Remedy

The exploration of herbal remedies in the context of brain cancer is a topic of growing interest, especially as many individuals seek complementary approaches to support their health during conventional cancer treatments. While scientific evidence supporting the efficacy of these remedies varies, some herbs have shown promise in preclinical studies or small clinical trials. Here's a more detailed look at some of the herbs previously mentioned and their potential roles:

1. Turmeric (Curcumin)-

Curcumin, the active compound in turmeric, is well-known for its anti-inflammatory and antioxidant properties. Research has suggested that curcumin may:

Inhibit Tumor Growth: Some studies indicate that curcumin can suppress the growth of various cancer cells, including glioblastoma cells, by inducing apoptosis (programmed cell death) and inhibiting cell proliferation.

Enhance Chemotherapy: Curcumin may enhance the effectiveness of certain chemotherapy drugs while potentially reducing their side effects.

2. Green Tea (Camellia sinensis): Green tea is rich in catechins, particularly EGCG, which has been studied for its potential anti-cancer effects:

Antioxidant Properties: The antioxidants in green tea may help protect cells from oxidative stress, which is a factor in cancer development.

Modulation of Signaling Pathways: EGCG may interfere with pathways involved in tumor growth and metastasis, making it a subject of interest in cancer research.

Ginseng (Panax ginseng): Ginseng has a long history of use in traditional medicine and is believed to have various health benefits:

Immune System Support: Ginseng may help boost immune function, which is important for cancer patients, especially during treatment.

Fatigue Reduction: Some studies suggest that ginseng can help reduce cancer-related fatigue, improving overall quality of life.

Milk Thistle (Silybum marianum): Milk thistle is primarily known for its liver-protective properties:

Liver Health: It may help mitigate liver damage caused by chemotherapy, potentially improving treatment tolerance.

Antioxidant Effects: Silymarin has antioxidant properties that may help reduce inflammation and support overall health.

Ginger (Zingiber officinale): Ginger is often used to manage nausea and digestive issues:

Nausea Relief: It is particularly effective in alleviating nausea caused by chemotherapy, making it a popular choice among cancer patients.

Anti-Inflammatory Properties: Ginger may help reduce inflammation, which is beneficial for overall health.

Ashwagandha (Withania somnifera): As an adaptogen, ashwagandha is thought to help the body adapt to stress:

Stress Reduction: It may help improve mental clarity and reduce anxiety, which can be especially important for cancer patients.

Potential Anti-Cancer Effects: Preliminary studies suggest it may have anti-cancer properties, though more research is needed.

Reishi Mushroom (Ganoderma lucidum): Reishi mushrooms have been used in traditional medicine for their health benefits:

Immune Modulation: Reishi may enhance immune function and has been studied for its potential anti-cancer effects.

Stress Relief: It may also have adaptogenic properties, helping to reduce stress.

Boswellia (Boswellia serrata): Boswellia, or frankincense, is recognized for its anti-inflammatory properties:

Anti-Inflammatory Effects: It may help reduce inflammation in the body, which is beneficial for cancer patients.

Potential Tumor Inhibition: Some studies suggest that boswellic acids may inhibit the growth of certain tumor types.

Holy Basil (Ocimum sanctum): Holy basil is valued for its adaptogenic and stress-relieving properties:

Immune Support: It may enhance immune function and help the body cope with the stress of illness.

Potential Anti-Cancer Effects: Some research indicates it may have properties that inhibit tumor growth.

Ginkgo Biloba: Ginkgo biloba is primarily known for its cognitive benefits:

Cognitive Function: It may help improve memory and cognitive function, which can be affected by brain cancer or its treatments.

Neuroprotective Properties: Some studies suggest ginkgo may have protective effects on brain cells.

While these herbs and natural products show potential as supportive therapies in the context of brain cancer, it is crucial to approach their use thoughtfully. Most importantly, patients should consult with their healthcare providers before starting any herbal regimen to ensure compatibility with their existing treatment plans and to avoid any adverse interactions. Research into the use of herbal remedies for cancer is ongoing, and while some studies provide encouraging results, more extensive clinical trials are needed to establish their efficacy and safety. Integrating herbal remedies with conventional treatment should always be part of a comprehensive care strategy tailored to individual needs and circumstances.

Herbal medicine for mesothelioma includes Essiac tea, astragalus, ginger, turmeric and others. It is used as a complementary therapy to ease cancer symptoms and relieve treatment side effects. Mesothelioma patients should consult their doctor before taking any herbal medicine.

Types of Herbs Used in Mesothelioma Treatment

Research suggests some herbal medicine may help people cope with cancer symptoms and side effects of cancer treatment. Research doesn't indicate herbal medicine can replace conventional cancer treatment. No herb has been proven to control or cure any kind of cancer.

Herbal medicine for mesothelioma includes Essiac tea, astragalus, ginger, turmeric and others. It is used as a complementary therapy to ease cancer symptoms and relieve treatment side effects. Mesothelioma patients should consult their doctor before taking any herbal medicine.

Types of Herbs Used in Mesothelioma Treatment

Research suggests some herbal medicine may help people cope with cancer symptoms and side effects of cancer treatment. Research doesn't indicate herbal medicine can replace conventional cancer treatment. No herb has been proven to control or cure any kind of cancer.

Research on Herbal Medicine for Cancer

Burdock Root: A 2011 review published in Inflammopharmacology discusses lab studies of burdock root that indicate the herb has anti-inflammatory, antibacterial, anti-cancer and liver-protecting properties. It hasn't been proven to treat cancer in humans, but it may reduce inflammation and help patients recover from liver damage after cancer treatment.

Essiac Tea: An herbal tea blend, it contains herbs known for their immune-boosting effects, including burdock root. Research shows Essiac tea doesn't cure cancer, but it does contain more antioxidants than red wine or green tea. The Memorial Sloan Kettering Cancer Center conducted about 18 studies on Essiac in the 1970s and 1980s. These studies found Essiac didn't boost the immune system or kill cancer cells.

Ginger: This herb shows anti-inflammatory and anti-cancer effects in lab studies. It can also reduce chemotherapy-related nausea and vomiting, according to a 2000 review published in the British Journal of Anaesthesia. But ginger should be strictly avoided before and after surgery. It promotes bleeding and patients with a low platelet count should avoid it.

Hypericin: This compound is found in St. John's Wort and it may help kill cancer cells. According to a 2000 study published in the Medical Journal of Australia, hypericin makes certain cancer cells more likely to die after photodynamic therapy, which is an experimental treatment for mesothelioma.

Moringa Tree: A 2006 test tube study published in the Journal of Experimental Therapeutics in Oncology found a compound in moringa tree effective at killing ovarian cancer cells. Other research suggests it may help cancer symptoms including difficulty breathing, cough, sore throat, fever and joint pain.

Cancer patients should exercise caution when using herbal products, as the quality control of these products may be inadequate. An example from the 1970s highlights the potential risks: A commercially available burdock root tea was discovered to be contaminated with atropine, a chemical known to cause irregular heartbeat and blurry vision. It's crucial for cancer patients to closely observe and assess the effects of any herbal remedies they consider using.

Free Mesothelioma Nutrition Guide

Eating the right diet throughout mesothelioma treatment can ease your symptoms.

Herbs for Treatment Side Effects
Several herbs may help control the side effects of conventional cancer treatment. For example, research done in humans suggests that mistletoe reduces the side effects of chemotherapy in lung cancer patients, and helps people with cancer tolerate higher doses of gemcitabine, which is used to treat mesothelioma.

Turmeric contains a compound know as curcumin, which research shows may be safe to combine with gemcitabine in cancer patients. It may also reduce bruising in surgery patients when combined with bromelain and arnica. Aloe vera taken during chemotherapy helped prevent mouth sores according to a review published in Cochrane Database Systematic Reviews.

Side Effect	Herbal Medicines
Nausea or vomiting	Ginger, Marijuana, Grape Seed, Peppermint, Roman Chamomile
Appetite loss	Marijuana, Dandelion, Devil's Claw, Lemon Balm, Siberian Ginseng
Diarrhea	Bilberry, Blackberry Leaf, Chamomile, Huanglian, Marshmallow Root
Constipation	Aloe Vera, Fenugreek, Ragweed, Senna, Psyllium
Fatigue	Astragalus, Chlorella, Ginkgo Biloba, Gotu Kola
Skin irritation	Calendula, Holy Basil, Milk Thistle, Panax Ginseng

Doctors don't recommend cancer patients take herbal medicine while undergoing cancer treatment. If you want to try herbal medicine during cancer treatment, talk to your oncologist about it so they can monitor your response and warn you of potential drug interactions. Some of these herbs might be safe to take after cancer treatment is completed, but you should get approval from your oncologist first.

According to studies, the herbs most commonly studied in cancer treatment include astragalus and dong quai. Much of the research has investigated these herbs in combination with chemotherapy.

Astragalus

Studies indicate astragalus may benefit lung cancer patients on chemotherapy.
Research on astragalus shows it may reduce the side effects of platinum-based chemotherapy agents such as cisplatin and carboplatin. These are two of the most effective chemotherapy drugs for mesothelioma.

A 2012 Chinese study published in Medical Oncology found improved quality of life among lung cancer patients who received a combination injection of astragalus, cisplatin and vinorelbine vs cisplatin and vinorelbine alone. The patients who received astragalus had better physical function and improved appetite. They also experienced less fatigue, pain, nausea and vomiting.

Make sure you discuss astragalus with your oncologist because it's a potent herb. It can alter the way your body processes chemotherapy in ways that may help or hurt depending on the patient.

Dong Quai
Traditional Chinese Medicine uses the herb dong quai to support overall wellness. The herb may offer additional benefits to cancer patients receiving doxorubicin, which is a chemotherapy drug used in the treatment of mesothelioma.

While there have been studies suggesting potential benefits of dong quai, it's important to note this herbal supplement can interact with certain medications and isn't recommended for women with estrogen-sensitive cancers. Furthermore, its safety for mesothelioma patients remains uncertain, and further clinical trials are needed to evaluate its effects.

One study published in 2007 in Basic and Clinical Pharmacology and Toxicology indicated dong quai may have a protective effect against the heart damage doxorubicin can cause. Additionally, a study published in 2006 in Oncology Reports suggested dong quai may offer protection against adiation therapy-induced lung inflammation.

Herbs for Cancer Symptoms
Certain herbal medicines may help mesothelioma cancer symptoms such

as pain and difficulty breathing. Some of these herbs have been studied in cancer patients, but some of them haven't.

Symptom	Herbal Medicines
Pain	Marijuana, Boswellia, Curcumin/Turmeric, White Willow Bark, Arnica
Shortness of breath	Hawthorn, Eucalyptus, Lobelia, White Pine Bark
Coughing	Black Cohosh, Slippery Elm Bark, White/Western Yarrow
Anxiety or stress	Kava, Passionflower, Magnolia Bark
Depression	St. John's Wort, Valerian
Sleeplessness or insomnia	Passionflower, Valerian, Chamomile

Because of the complexities of interactions and the specific considerations for different cancer types, mesothelioma patients must consult with their health care providers before considering the use of any herbal supplement. They can advise when it may be safe to take supplements and warn you about potential drug interactions.

How Does Herbal Medicine Work for Cancer?

Clinical trials that combine herbal medicine with cancer therapies are relatively new to the United States. China has performed such trials since the early 1900s. Cancer doctors rely on clinical trials to recommend treatments that are proven effective. The lack of clinical trials on herbal medicines has limited what doctors can safely recommend.

Herbs may seem harmless, but sometimes they can interfere with cancer treatment. For example, some herbs can prevent chemotherapy and radiation therapy from killing cancer cells. Certain herbs enhance the effect of chemotherapy in a toxic way that leads to unwanted side effects.

Herbal medicine may come in the form of tablets or capsules, creams, teas or tinctures (an alcohol-based concentrate). Doctors recommend patients avoid herbs during treatment. It won't be safe until research can identify which herbs are safe to combine with cancer treatment. People with cancer should get approval from their oncologist first before they take any kind of herbal medicine because some herbs may negatively impact the outcome of cancer treatment.

Is Herbal Medicine Effective and Safe for Mesothelioma?

In general, herbal medicines aren't as effective as conventional medicine for mesothelioma. While some people feel relief from herbal medicine for mild symptoms or side effects, many people get more relief from prescription medication.

Studies conducted in test tubes and animals have shown some anti-cancer effects of various herbs, but these results haven't been replicated in human trials. Research on other herbs has also shown a mix of benefits and risks for people with cancer. For example, some herbs promote bleeding with surgery, block the body's removal of cancer drugs or increase their toxicity. delaying the metabolism of certain drugs.

Potential Benefits of Herbs
Boost the immune system
Ease cancer symptoms
Reduce treatment side effects
Slow cancer spreading (metastasis)
Attack cancer cells
The U.S. Food and Drug Administration designates most herbs as GRAS, or generally recognized as safe. They often have a lower risk of side effects

because they're less potent than pharmaceuticals. Constipation is the most common side effect. However, herbal remedies are still a type of medicine. Make sure to get approval first from your oncologist.

Research in a developing field of medicine known as integrative oncology attempts to understand which complementary therapies, including herbal medicines, are safe and effective to combine with conventional cancer treatments. Most of the research has been conducted in test tube studies or mouse studies. Some research involving humans has been conducted internationally, but no large, double-blind controlled clinical trials have been conducted in the U.S.

Consult Your Doctor About Herbal Medicine

The importance of discussing herbal remedies with your oncologist before buying or trying them can't be stressed enough. All too often patients don't discuss the supplements and herbs they want to take with their doctor first.

Your oncologist has your best interest at heart and only wants to protect you from potentially harmful interactions. In many cases, your doctor will give their approval to take herbal remedies after you complete treatment.

A common misconception is that natural products can't be harmful or that they're always safe to combine with pharmaceutical medications. Many natural substances such as arsenic and tobacco are poisonous and carcinogenic. The effects of herbs can range from mild to potent depending on the person taking them and the medications they're using.

It's wise to thoroughly research the herbs you want to try and take your research to your oncologist. This allows your doctor to advise you with as much information as possible.

In summary, Brain cancer refers to malignant tumors that develop in the brain or central nervous system. It can be classified into primary brain tumors, which originate from brain tissue, and secondary (metastatic) brain tumors, which spread to the brain from other parts of the body.

Common types of brain cancer include: - Gliomas[Tumors from glial cells, including astrocytomas (with glioblastoma being the most aggressive), oligodendrogliomas, and ependymomas.], Meningiomas[Usually benign tumors arising from the meninges, the protective membranes around the brain.], Acoustic Neuromas[Benign tumors affecting the vestibular nerve, leading to hearing loss and balance issues.], Medulloblastomas[Aggressive tumors primarily found in children, often located in the cerebellum.], Pituitary Tumors[Tumors from the pituitary gland that can affect hormone levels.]

Symptoms may vary but commonly include persistent headaches, seizures, nausea, cognitive changes, and sensory disturbances.

Diagnosis typically involves medical history review, neurological examination, imaging studies like MRI or CT scans, and sometimes a biopsy to confirm the tumor type.

Treatment approaches may include: - Surgery(To remove the tumor or obtain tissue samples.), Radiation Therapy(To target and kill cancer cells, often used post-surgery.), Chemotherapy(Systemic treatment to inhibit tumor growth.), Targeted Therapy and Immunotherapy(Emerging options focused on specific tumor characteristics or enhancing the immune response.)

The prognosis for brain cancer varies widely based on tumor type, location, and response to treatment. Some tumors have favorable outcomes, while others remain challenging to treat.

Brain cancer is a complex and serious condition requiring comprehensive care. Advances in research are continually improving diagnosis and treatment options, offering hope for better patient outcomes.

Printed in Great Britain
by Amazon